the pocket glucose revolution
and sports nutrition

DR HELEN O'CONNOR • DR JENNIE BRAND MILLER
DR STEPHEN COLAGIURI • KAYE FOSTER-POWELL

CORONET BOOKS
Hodder & Stoughton

Copyright © 1997 by Helen O'Connor, Janette Brand Miller,
Kaye Foster-Powell and Dr Stephen Colagiuri

The right of Helen O'Connor, Janette Brand Miller, Kaye Foster-Powell and Dr Stephen Colagiuri to be identified as the Authors of the Work has been asserted by them in accordance with the Copyright, Designs and Patents Act 1988.

First published in Australia in 1997 by
Hodder Headline Australia Pty Limited

First published in Great Britain in 2000
by Hodder and Stoughton
A division of Hodder Headline

This United Kingdom edition is published by arrangement with
Hodder Headline Australia Pty Limited
A Coronet Paperback

10 9 8 7 6 5 4 3 2 1

All rights reserved. No part of this publication may be reproduced, stored in a retrieval system, or transmitted, in any form or by any means without the prior written permission of the publisher, nor be otherwise circulated in any form of binding or cover other than that in which it is published and without a similar condition being imposed on the subsequent purchaser.

A CIP catalogue record for this title is available from the
British Library

ISBN 0 340 76988 2

Printed and bound in Great Britain by
Omnia Books Ltd, Glasgow

Hodder and Stoughton
A division of Hodder Headline
338 Euston Road
London NW1 3BH

CONTENTS

Introduction	5
Is your diet fit for peak performance?	6
Sports nutrition in a nutshell	9
Are you really choosing low fat?	11
Sources of iron	14
Energy charge your body with carbohydrate	18
3 steps to estimate your daily carbohydrate needs	20
What's your activity level?	21
Jessica's carbohydrate needs	22
Jessica's typical daily diet	22
Which carbohydrate foods are best?	24
What is the G.I. factor?	25
Understanding the G.I. factor	26
How the G.I. is measured	27
Is there an easy way to tell if a food has a high or low G.I.?	30
Tricky twins	31
How can I calculate the G.I. of a mixed meal?	32
How can I use the G.I. to boost sports performance?	33
The case for high G.I. foods	34
Recovery after exercise	34
Table 1: Serving sizes of high G.I. foods to enhance recovery	37
During an event	38
Table 2: High G.I. choices suitable during exercise	39
Eating for competing: carbohydrate loading-what a load of glycogen!	42
Do you need to carbohydrate load?	43
What about the G.I. and carbohydrate loading?	43
The pre-competition meal	44
On your mark...get set...go	45
The case for low G.I. foods	46

The pre-event meal	46
Weight control	48
Counting the Calories in our nutrients	49
The case studies	50
Nathan – Australian Rules football	51
Meal plan for Nathan	54
Analise – ballet dancer	56
Meal plan for Analise	60
Ian – ironman triathlete	62
Meal plan for Ian	67
The pre-event meal plan for Ian	69
Your G.I. questions answered	70
How to use the G.I. tables	72
A–Z of foods with G.I. factor, carbohydrate & fat	74
How to find a sports dietitian	94
Recommended reading on sports nutrition	95
About the authors	96

INTRODUCTION

Sports nutrition is a new and dynamic science dedicated to unravelling the key nutrition factors that boost sports performance. What you eat does make a difference to your performance. The trick is getting into the right eating routine, keeping up to date and ignoring the confusing nutrition myths that abound.

This book looks at a new key factor: the G.I. factor. Australian researchers were the first to see the potential in applying the G.I. factor to athletes' diets to enhance sports performance. This guide shows you how to use the G.I. factor in your own diet to boost your sports performance. When you pop this pocket book into your training bag, you'll have:

- a quick quiz to help you assess your current eating habits
- refuelling hints at your fingertips
- case studies that provide you with fun, easy and practical ways to eat your way to better performance
- G.I. tables of foods including sports drinks plus their fat and carbohydrate count

What you eat does make a difference to your sports performance.

IS YOUR DIET FIT FOR PEAK PERFORMANCE?

Take the diet fitness quiz and see how well you score. It's a good idea to use this quiz regularly to pick up on areas where you may need to improve your diet.

1. Circle your answer.

Eating patterns

■ I eat at least 3 meals a day with no longer than 5 hours in between   Yes/No

---

Carbohydrate checker

■ I eat at least 4 slices of bread (or alternatives) each day (1 roll = 2 slices of bread, ½ cup rice, 1 potato)   Yes/No

■ I eat at least 1 cup of breakfast cereal each day or an extra slice of bread   Yes/No

■ I usually eat 2 or more pieces of fruit each day   Yes/No

■ I eat at least 3 different vegetables or have a salad most days   Yes/No

■ I include carbohydrates like pasta, rice and potato in my diet each day   Yes/No

---

Protein checker

■ I eat at least 1 and usually 2 servings of meat or meat alternatives (poultry, seafood, eggs, dried peas/beans or nuts) each day   Yes/No

Fat checker

- I spread butter or margarine thinly on bread or use none at all — Yes/No
- I eat fried food no more than once per week — Yes/No
- I use polyunsaturated or mono-unsaturated oil (e.g. olive oil) for cooking. (Circle yes if you never fry in oil or fat) — Yes/No
- I avoid oil-based dressings on salads — Yes/No
- I use reduced fat or low fat dairy products — Yes/No
- I cut the fat off meat and take the skin off chicken — Yes/No
- I eat fatty snacks such as chocolate, chips, biscuits, rich desserts, cakes, pies and pastries no more than twice a week — Yes/No
- I eat fast or take-away food no more than once per week — Yes/No

....

Iron checker

- I eat lean red meat at least 3 times per week or 2 servings of white meat daily or for vegetarians, include at least 1–2 cups of dried peas and beans (e.g. lentils, soy beans, chick peas) daily — Yes/No
- I include a vitamin C source with meals based on bread, cereals, fruit and vegetables to assist the iron absorption in these 'plant' sources of iron — Yes/No

Calcium checker
■ I eat at least 3 servings of dairy food or soy milk alternative each day (1 serving = 200 ml milk or fortified soy milk; 1 slice (30 g) hard cheese; 200 g yoghurt)   Yes/No

Fluids
■ I drink fluids regularly before, during and after exercise   Yes/No

Alcohol
■ When I drink alcohol, I would mostly drink no more than is recommended for the safe drink driving limit   Yes/No
(Circle yes if you don't drink alcohol)

2. Score 1 point for every 'yes' answer

Scoring scale
18–20 Excellent   15–17 Room for improvement
12–14 just made it   0–12 Poor

Note: Very active people will need to eat more breads, cereals and fruit than on this quiz, but to stay healthy no one should be eating less.

(Adapted from *The Taste of Fitness* by Helen O'Connor and Donna Hay)

SPORTS NUTRITION IN A NUTSHELL
High carbohydrate eating
To perform at its best, your body needs the right type of fuel. No matter what your sport, carbohydrates are the best fuel for you! High carbohydrate foods help enhance stamina and prevent fatigue. They include, breakfast cereals, bread, rice, pasta, fruit and vegetables (especially starchy vegetables like potato, corn and dried peas and beans). Sugars found in table sugar, honey, jam and confectionery are also useful sources of carbohydrate for active people.

Low fat eating
Fats are an essential part of your diet. A low to moderate fat intake helps active people maintain a lean physique. Eating the best types of fat and avoiding excessive fat intake is important for good health and optional performance. The best types of fats for cooking include the mono-unsaturated fats like olive oil and the poly-unsaturated fats like sunflower and safflower oil. Watch out for the saturated fats found in many fast foods, butter, cream and the fat on meat.

Fat reducing strategies include:

- cutting the fat off meat (or using trim cuts)
- removing the skin from chicken
- using minimal amounts of fat in cooking
- using non-stick cookware

The amount of fat you need depends on your daily fuel requirements. For good health and weight maintenance we have included the following general guidelines. (5 g fat is equivalent to about 1 teaspoon mono- or polyunsaturated oil.)

- Low fat diets — 30–40 g fat per day
- Most women and children — 30–50 g fat per day
- Most men — 40–60 g fat per day
- Teenagers and active adults — 70 g fat per day
- Larger and very active athletes/workers — 80–100 g fat per day

Fat is an 'invisible' ingredient in many foods. Use a fat counter to help you identify some of the sources of fat in your diet. Keep a food record for a week and calculate your personal fat intake using the counter. It may surprise you! Comprehensive fat counters are readily available from bookshops and newsagents. We have also included a fat counter in the A–Z of Foods tables in this pocket guide starting on page 74.

ARE YOU REALLY CHOOSING LOW FAT?

There's a trick to food labels that it is worth being aware of when shopping for low fat foods. Nutrient claims are covered by food legislation that specifies what low fat really means.

Low fat means that the food must be 5% fat or less (5 g fat per 100 g food).

Reduced fat means that the food contains at least 25% less fat than the original food – in other words, no more than 75% of the fat found in the original food. A reduced fat food isn't low enough in fat to be called a low fat food.

A balanced diet contains a wide variety of low fat foods.

Don't forget protein
Athletes in heavy training have increased protein needs. Protein balance depends on the individual but you generally need at least 2 servings a day. Some athletes forget to include enough protein in their diet (2–3 servings per day). Body building athletes often consume protein in excess of their requirements. Good sources of protein include lean meat, poultry, fish and seafood, eggs, milk, cheese and yoghurt. Dried peas, beans and nuts are the best vegetable source. Bread and cereals provide smaller but still useful amounts of protein.

Fluids
The human body is 70 per cent water. During exercise you lose some of this water as sweat. If you don't replace it, you will become dehydrated and your body will overheat – like a car without water in its radiator.

- Small fluid losses decrease mental and physical performance.
- Large fluid losses resulting in dehydration are life threatening!

During exercise, thirst is not a good indicator of your fluid needs. You usually need to drink more than your thirst dictates. Every kilogram lost during exercise approximates 1 litre of sweat losses to be replaced.

*During exercise,
thirst is not a good indicator
of your fluid needs.*

What to drink during exercise
Water is an adequate fluid replacer and is appropriate in many situations.
Sports and electrolyte drinks are absorbed into the bloodstream faster than water, replace carbohydrates and electrolytes and have a pleasant taste—which encourages greater fluid consumption. See 'The Case for High G.I. Foods' (pages 34–41) for more on sports drinks. The A–Z of Foods (page 93) gives the G.I. of sports drinks, such as Gatorade.
Soft drinks or fruit juice empty from the stomach slower than sports drinks or water and aren't suitable fluid replacers during exercise.
Note: The caffeine in cola-type soft drinks increases urine production and is dehydrating.

*Adequate fluid replacement
during exercise enhances performance
and prevents heat stress.*

Special nutrient considerations

Iron Iron deficiency is common in athletes, particularly female athletes, vegetarians, and those participating in strenuous training programs, especially endurance athletes. Many athletes don't consume adequate iron in their daily diet and may include excess caffeine or tannin (in tea) that bind up iron and reduce its absorption. The best sources of iron are red meats, liver and kidney. Plant sources contain lower amounts of iron which is not absorbed as well. The iron in iron supplements is also less well absorbed than the iron in red meat.

SOURCES OF IRON
(ranked from best to least):

- ******** Red meats, liver, kidney
- ******* White meats and seafood
- ****** Dried peas and beans (baked beans, soy beans)
- ***** Bread, cereals and some vegetables

Did you know?

Including vitamin C rich fruits and vegetables in a meal improves the absorption or iron from plant sources (e.g. bread, cereals, vegetables, fruit). Drinking a glass of orange juice with your breakfast cereal in the morning will increase the amount of iron absorbed from this meal.

Calcium Calcium is important for bone development in the young and for bone maintenance in adults. An adequate calcium intake and weight-bearing exercise throughout life is essential to build and then maintain optimal bone strength for both males and females.

> *Calcium is important*
> *for bone development in the young*
> *and for bone maintenance in adults.*

In females, regular strenuous exercise, usually accompanied by factors such as fat loss, strict dieting or stress, can precipitate menstrual cycle interruptions. An irregular or absent menstrual cycle may result in a reduced level of the hormone oestrogen which is vital for maintaining calcium levels in bone and for enhancing calcium absorption from the diet. Menstrual irregularities of greater than six months need medical investigation. Athletes with very infrequent or absent menstrual cycles should have extra calcium in the range of 1000 to 1500 mg a day. This won't prevent bone loss but may help to slow down the rate of loss.

Nutritional supplements
Big dollars are spent promoting nutritional supplements for active people and athletes. Watch out for supplements with no scientific basis to the claims. If in doubt, ask a sports dietitian for help. Some supplements are beneficial in certain circumstances.

Supplements of iron or calcium may be required if inadequate amounts are consumed in the diet or if deficiency exists.

Supplements like sports drinks, liquid meals and carbohydrate loaders are also beneficial, not because they provide something magical but because they package energy and carbohydrate in a convenient and easy to consume form. This is especially useful to athletes who need an easily digested fuel on the run.

Sports bars and carbohydrate gels (available in sports and bike shops) are in a similar category to sports drinks etc.

Herbal supplements, amino acids and fat burners
Unfortunately, solid evidence for these supplements is lacking. In many cases, scientific studies have shown that they have absolutely no effect on fat loss, muscle enlargement or performance.

Competition eating

Eating for competing is discussed in detail later in this book. Look under the following topics:

- pre-competition meal guidelines (page 44)
- the case for low G.I. foods (page 46)
- glycogen loading (page 42)
- recovery after exercise (page 34)
- the case for high G.I. foods (page 34)
- refuelling during an event (page 38)

If you want to find out about eating for competing in greater depth, take a look at one of the books on sports nutrition in the references on page 95 or consult a sports dietitian.

*Whether you are one of the elite
or a weekend warrior,
the right diet can give you
the winning edge.*

ENERGY CHARGE YOUR BODY WITH CARBOHYDRATE

Carbohydrate circulates in your body as glucose in the blood (blood sugar) and is stored as glycogen in the liver and muscles. Your body uses glucose to fuel movement and activity. Just as high speed cars require regular top-ups of petrol, active bodies need a regular supply of carbohydrate to top up glycogen stores. When glycogen stores are depleted, fatigue sets in and performance suffers.

Carbohydrate is the human body's main energy source for physical activity, especially high intensity exercise.

But your body's carbohydrate stores are small, and need regular replenishing, generally every 4 to 5 hours. Athletes feel tired and lethargic when they don't consume enough carbohydrate for their daily needs. When this happens and the glycogen in the muscles is depleted, fatigue sets in. That's when your muscles feel heavy and your pace slows. 'Hitting the wall', an expression used by endurance athletes, refers to the feeling when glycogen stores are almost exhausted.

Active bodies need a regular supply of carbohydrate to top up on their glycogen stores.

Low blood sugar or 'hypoglycaemia'
Exercisers can also experience a type of fatigue related to the carbohydrate levels in their blood. It is possible for your muscle glycogen levels to be adequate while the blood sugar levels controlled by the liver, fall. Low blood sugar or 'hypoglycaemia' occurs when you exercise in the morning before eating, or exercise hard after skipping a meal.

> *To maintain energy levels,*
> *athletes must consume enough carbohydrate*
> *to keep pace with their muscle glycogen needs*
> *and keep up a regular intake of carbohydrate*
> *to maintain blood sugar levels.*

Early morning exercise
If you exercise strenuously early in the morning, it's a good idea to have some carbohydrate before training or take some with you to have on the run! Most people have enough liver glycogen to fuel low intensity, short duration (<1 hour) exercise sessions. If you simply want to delay eating until after your light early morning walk, it's not a problem. However, eating before and/or during a strenuous cycling session makes good sense!

3 EASY STEPS TO ESTIMATE YOUR DAILY CARBOHYDRATE NEEDS

It is difficult to put an exact figure on anyone's carbohydrate needs. Use the table opposite as a rough guide and ask a sports dietitian for help if you are unsure.

Step 1. Weigh yourself naked or in minimal clothing in kilograms (no shoes or belts with heavy buckles!).

Step 2. Multiply your body weight by your activity level factor (see table opposite). This total gives you the **target carbohydrate intake in grams** that you must consume each day to meet your carbohydrate needs.

Step 3. Keep a food record for a few days and calculate your carbohydrate intake with a carbohydrate counter such as the one at the end of this book. Compare your actual carbohydrate intake with the target value you calculated. If it is way below the carbohydrate target, you have some serious carb eating to do! If you are within 50 g or even a little over your carbohydrate target that's fine! Use the carbohydrate counter to help you plan a higher carb intake.

Remember, this is a rough estimate.
You may need a little more or less.
See how you feel.

WHAT'S YOUR ACTIVITY LEVEL?

The amount of carbohydrate you need depends on your weight and activity level.

Activity level	Grams of carbohydrate per kg body weight per day
Light – Walking, light/easy swimming or cycling low impact/easy beat aerobic dance *Less than 1 hour per day*	4–5
Light-moderate – intermediate aerobic dance class, easy jog, non-competitive tennis (3 sets), netball *1 hour per day*	5–6
Moderate – 1 hour run, serious training for recreational/competition sports such as soccer, basketball, squash *1–2 hours per day*	6–7
Moderate-heavy – most professional/elite training for competitive sport such as swimming, tennis, football, distance running (<marathon) *2–4 hours per day*	7–8
Heavy – Training for ironman events marathon running/swimming, Olympic distance triathlon *More than 4 hours per day*	8–10

■ Activity levels refer to the intensity as well as the duration of the activity.
■ Time refers to the amount of time you are physically active during training, not the amount of time at training.
■ Body weight refers to ideal or 'healthy' body weight.

JESSICA'S CARBOHYDRATE NEEDS

Step 1. Weight 58 kg

Step 2. Activity Moderate level (training for mid-distance fun runs – recreational level)
Requires 6–7 g of carbohydrate per kilogram per day
Target carbohydrate level is
6 × 58 = 348 g per day to 7 × 58 = 406 g per day
348–406 g per day

Step 3. Food record

JESSICA'S FOOD RECORD

Meal	Carbohydrate count (g)
Breakfast	
1 cup of bran cereal	35
½ cup of milk	5
1 slice of white toast with butter	15
150 ml no added sugar fruit juice	15
Snack	
1 banana	32
Lunch	
1 cheese and tomato sandwich on white bread	32
1 low fat fruit yoghurt	26
1 glass water	0

Snack

2 cracker biscuits with Marmite	12
1 orange	10

Dinner

1 small piece of steak	0
1 medium potato	16
½ cup of mixed vegetables	7
2 small scoops reduced fat ice-cream	13

Supper

3 plain coffee biscuits	14

Total carbohydrate — 225

Jessica's carbohydrate count is way below target.
To boost Jessica's carbohydrate intake, add:

1 extra piece of toast at breakfast	15
1 extra sandwich and fruit or juice at lunch	45
1 cup cooked pasta or rice with dinner	55
1 bread roll with dinner	30
1 glass of hot milk at supper	7

Grand total boosted with the extra carbohydrate foods — 377 g

This is in the middle of the recommended range for Jessica's weight and activity level. Depending on how she feels, slight adjustments may be required depending on variations in the intensity and duration of her training program.

WHICH CARBOHYDRATE FOODS ARE BEST?

Carbohydrate foods include breads, breakfast cereals, rice and pasta, fruit and vegetables, especially starchy vegetables like potato, corn and dried peas and beans. There are smaller amounts of carbohydrate in dairy foods and in processed foods containing sugars. The carbohydrate foods give you a range of nutrients essential for health. When you are establishing the overall balance of your diet it is important to consume more of the carbohydrate foods which contain a high proportion of nutrients rather than those without additional vitamins and minerals.

Many active people, especially athletes in heavy training who eat large volumes of food, easily meet their daily nutrient requirements. Their carbohydrate needs, however, are sometimes so high, they simply can't manage the volume they need to eat! Liquid meals or carbohydrate supplements can help these athletes with high energy requirements meet their energy needs in a less 'bulky' way.

Today, there's another vital consideration in selecting carbohydrate foods to boost your sports performance. It is the glycaemic index of a food – the G.I. factor.

WHAT IS THE G.I. FACTOR?

Research on the glycaemic index (what we call the G.I. factor) shows that different carbohydrate foods have dramatically different effects on blood sugar levels.

The G.I. factor ranks foods based on their immediate effect on your blood sugar levels.

The carbohydrate score board

The G.I. ranking of carbohydrate foods is similar to a point score ranking in sports performance. The fastest athlete scoring the most points goes to the top, the slowest scorer is ranked at the bottom. The G.I. ranks carbohydrate foods on the speed at which they enter the bloodstream. The faster a blood sugar response appears in the bloodstream after eating a food, the higher its ranking or its G.I. The longer it takes to observe a blood sugar response, the lower the G.I.

At the 'back of the pack' of carbohydrate foods are legumes e.g. soy beans, baked beans, lentils etc. These enter the bloodstream slowly and have a very low G.I. (soy beans have a G.I. between 14–18).

UNDERSTANDING THE G.I. FACTOR

The glycaemic index concept was first developed by Dr David Jenkins, a professor of nutrition at the University of Toronto, Canada, to help determine which foods were best for people with diabetes. Since then, scientists around the world, including the authors of this book, have tested the effect of many foods on blood sugar levels and clearly demonstrated the value of the glycaemic index.

The key is the rate of digestion

Carbohydrate foods that break down quickly during digestion have the highest G.I. factors. Conversely, carbohydrates which break down slowly, releasing glucose gradually into the bloodstream have low G.I. factors.

Low G.I.	**less than 55**
Intermediate G.I.	**55 to 70**
High G.I.	**more than 70**

HOW THE G.I. IS MEASURED?

You can't predict the G.I. of a food from its composition. To test the G.I., you need real people and real foods. Standardised methods are always followed so that scientists around the world can duplicate the tests and the results from one group of people can be directly compared with those from another. The glycaemic response to a test food is determined by measuring the rise in blood sugar level and monitoring how long this level stays elevated.

Pure glucose produces the greatest rise in blood sugar levels. All other foods have less effect when fed in equal amounts of carbohydrate. The G.I. of pure glucose is set at 100 and every other food is ranked on a scale from 0 to 100 according to its actual effect on blood sugar levels.

You can't predict the G.I. of a food from its composition

1. To find out the G.I. of a food, a volunteer eats an amount of that food containing 50 g of carbohydrate (calculated from food composition tables) – 50 g of carbohydrate is equivalent to 3 tablespoons of pure glucose powder.
2. Over the next 2 hours (3 hours if the volunteer has diabetes), a blood sample is taken every 15 minutes during the first hour and every 30 minutes thereafter and the blood sugar level of these samples is measured and recorded.
3. The blood sugar level is plotted on a graph and the area under the curve is calculated using a computer program (see Figure 1).
4. The volunteer's response to the test food is compared with his or her blood sugar response to 50 g of pure glucose (the reference food).
5. The reference food is tested on 2 or 3 separate occasions and an average value is calculated to reduce the effect of day-to-day variation in blood sugar responses.

Note: The G.I. factor of the test food is the average value of a group of 8 to 12 volunteers.

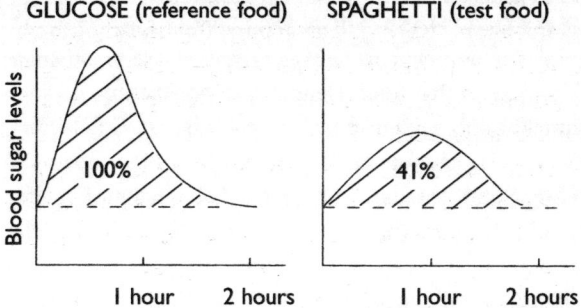

Figure 1. The effect of a food on blood sugar levels is calculated using the area under the curve (hatched area). The area under the curve after consumption of the test food is compared with the same area after the reference food (usually 50 g of pure glucose or a 50 g carbohydrate portion of white bread).

Take some time to browse through the G.I. tables at the back of this book. Some of the G.I. factors may surprise you! At first it is hard to believe that sugar-containing foods may have a lower G.I. to fibrous, starchy foods like potato. But remember, these blood sugar responses have been measured numerous times and the tests have been repeated by different scientists around the world.

IS THERE AN EASY WAY TO TELL IF A FOOD HAS A HIGH OR LOW G.I.?

No! The only way to tell is to measure the blood sugar response to that food. Generally, foods that break down quickly during digestion have the highest G.I. factors. The G.I. cannot be predicted from the chemical composition of the food or the G.I. factor of related foods. Milling and grinding break down the cellular structure of grains and tend to speed up the rate of digestion, which increases the G.I. Cooking increases the digestibility of starch, and may also increase the G.I. It might seem surprising but removing the dietary fibre in bread, rice or pasta has little effect on the G.I. However, the viscous fibre found in fruits and some grains (e.g. oats and barley) may account for their lower G.I. Fat slows the digestion process and lowers the G.I. in some instances.

The only way to tell if a food has a high or low G.I. is to measure it.

TRICKY TWINS

Circle the food in each of the following pairs which you think will have the lower G.I. factor.

Rice	Rice Krispies
Sweet corn	Cornflakes
Baked potatoes	French fries
Toasted muesli	Untoasted muesli
Grainy bread	Wholemeal bread

(Answers: Rice, Sweet corn, Baked potatoes, Toasted muesli, Grainy bread – depending on the brand.)

HOW CAN I CALCULATE THE G.I. OF A MIXED MEAL?

You calculate the G.I. of a mixed meal by averaging the G.I. of the different carbohydrate foods in the meal. Supposing you have baked beans on toast, both of which are carbohydrate foods.

Regular white bread has a G.I. of 70 and baked beans have a G.I. of 48. If equal amounts of carbohydrate come from the baked beans and the bread then you add the G.I. factors and divide by two, e.g. $(70 + 48)/2 = 59$.

Say the meal contained one-quarter of the carbohydrate from baked beans to three-quarters of the carbohydrate from bread then 25 per cent of the G.I. factor for baked beans would be added to 75 per cent of the G.I. for bread. The following calculation shows how this is done.

$$\begin{aligned} 25 \text{ per cent of } 48 &= 12 \\ 75 \text{ per cent of } 70 &= 52.5 \\ \text{G.I. factor} &= 12 + 52.5 = 64.5 \end{aligned}$$

But you really don't need to do calculations. All you need to remember is:

Low G.I. + High G.I. = Intermediate G.I.

HOW CAN I USE THE G.I. TO BOOST SPORTS PERFORMANCE?

There are several applications of the G.I. to sports performance. Sometimes it will be best for you to choose a high G.I. food, other times, a low G.I. food may be beneficial.

To date, most work on the G.I. factor and sports performance has concentrated on competition eating and recovery. Researchers are investigating other applications, especially the G.I. at each meal over the day when athletes are undergoing different training programs and exercise intensities. Scientific research has so far identified three key applications of the G.I. to enhance performance.

1. High G.I. foods in the recovery phase after exercise to accelerate glycogen replenishment.
2. High G.I. foods or fluids during exercise to maintain blood sugar levels.
3. A low G.I. pre-event meal may enhance endurance in prolonged exercise.

THE CASE FOR HIGH G.I. FOODS

RECOVERY AFTER EXERCISE

After exercise, your muscles are hungry for carbohydrate. Postponing carbohydrate consumption after exercise delays muscle glycogen replenishment and can cause fatigue.

- If you are a recreational exerciser, an adequate carbohydrate intake over the next few days will ensure that muscles are ready for another session.
- If you are participating in strenuous training, particularly when two or more training sessions are part of the daily routine, rapid glycogen replenishment is vital. Eat or drink carbohydrate (within 30 minutes) after strenuous exercise when another training session is on the agenda a few hours later. On consecutive days of competition, this recovery strategy will also assist in restocking your glycogen stores for the next event.

In the immediate post exercise period, high G.I. carbohydrates are best because they are digested and absorbed much faster and stimulate more insulin – the hormone responsible for getting glucose into the muscle and storing it as glycogen. Most athletes prefer high carbohydrate drinks because they are usually thirsty rather than hungry after strenuous exercise. A drink also aids rehydration.

Sports or electrolyte replacement drinks are ideal for replacing fluids and providing an immediate and convenient source of high G.I. carbohydrate.

After this initial 'hit' of recovery carbs, try to make sure your next meal or snack (within 2 hours) includes intermediate to high G.I. foods.

Recovery formula
The amount of carbohydrate required to kick off the recovery process is about 1 g per kilogram of body weight. Most people need between 50 to 100 grams of carbohydrate in the immediate post exercise period. Table 1 outlines a list of convenient high G.I. foods and sports drinks, suitable for recovery.

> *Postponing carbohydrate consumption after exercise delays muscle glycogen replenishment and can cause fatigue.*

TABLE 1: SERVING SIZES OF HIGH G.I. FOODS TO ENHANCE RECOVERY

Food	G.I.	Serving size = 50 grams carbohydrate	Serving size = 75 grams carbohydrate
White or brown bread	70	100 grams (3 slices)	150 grams (4–5 slices)
Rice Krispies (Kelloggs)	89	45 grams (1½ cups + 175 ml milk)	65 grams (2 cups + 300 ml milk)
Cornflakes (Kelloggs)	84	45 grams (1½ cups + 175 ml milk)	65 grams (2 cups + 300 ml milk)
Scones	70	150 grams (2 large scones)	200 grams (3 large scones)
Morning coffee biscuits	79	65 grams (10 biscuits)	100 grams (15 biscuits)
Rice cakes	82	60 grams (5 rice cakes)	90 grams (8 rice cakes)
Muffins (toasted)	70	120 grams (2 muffins)	180 grams (3 muffins)
Rice, cooked	83	180 grams (1 cup)	270 grams (1½ cups)

Food	G.I.	Serving size = 50 grams carbohydrate	Serving size = 75 grams carbohydrate
Jelly beans	80	54 grams (6 jelly beans)	81 grams (9 jelly beans)
Sports electrolyte drink 6% carb	73–78	850 ml	1250 ml

Females weighing about 50 kilograms should aim to eat 50 grams of carbohydrate.

Males weighing about 75 kilograms should aim to eat 75 grams of carbohydrate.

DURING AN EVENT

High G.I. carbohydrate is the best choice to optimise performance as the carbohydrate needs to be rapidly available to the muscle as a fuel source. Consuming carbohydrate 'on the run' has been shown to delay fatigue as it provides energy to working muscles when the body's own stores of glycogen are low. This is especially the case when exercise is prolonged and even glycogen loading cannot prepare the body for the carbohydrate needed to get through the long endurance event.

If you don't have sufficient carbohydrate in your training diet, supplementing carbohydrate during exercise helps you keep pace when your glycogen stores are low. This is not a quick fix to avoid a high carbohydrate training diet! The body prefers to obtain carbs from glycogen stored in the muscle during exercise. Outside carbs are a great back up, but it's essential to prepare your body by eating a high carb training diet each day.

Table 2 lists high G.I. carbohydrates that are popular during exercise. Sports electrolyte replacement drinks are usually tolerated better because they are emptied more quickly from the stomach.

TABLE 2: HIGH G.I. CHOICES SUITABLE DURING EXERCISE

Food	G.I.	Serving size	Carbohydrate (g)
Sport drink (electrolyte)	73–78	1 litre	60–80
White bread with honey	70	2 slices with 2 tsp honey	40
Breakfast bar (fruit flavour)	78	1 bar	29
Jelly beans	80	100 g	60
Rice cakes	82	5 cakes	50
Scones	70	2 large	50

Prolong your endurance by topping up fluids and carbohydrate regularly throughout exercise.

Sports or electrolyte replacement drinks are ideal as they encourage greater fluid consumption than water, enhance intestinal absorption of fluid and provide carbohydrate while rehydrating the body at the same time. They are also less likely to cause gastrointestinal distress than solid foods. Getting the tummy wobbles during competition is not desirable!

The choice of solid or liquid carbohydrate during exercise is ultimately up to the individual, however, with the current sports/electrolyte formulations providing an optimal quickly absorbed source of carbs, it is hard to look past this as a primary option. Many exercisers choose a combination of sports drinks and comfortable solid foods they have trialled in training. Solids help in prolonged exercise to fill that 'empty' feeling in the stomach.

Many of the popular foods used during exercise over the years were adopted because they were convenient or easy to eat, rather than because they had a high G.I. The ever popular banana for example has an intermediate G.I. Eating a banana during exercise is not wrong. However, when the pace is really on and you want a fast energy supply, a more rapidly absorbing high G.I. option would technically be better. In prolonged exercise, you should aim to consume 30–60 g of carbohydrate per hour over the session (or event).

In long events, a combination of comfortable foods whatever their G.I. along with the high G.I. options will provide the best variety and feeling of psychological well being. The occasional mini chocolate bar as a treat may not scientifically be the best, highest G.I. fuel during exercise, but in the final stages of the ironman, it may boost your morale enough to keep you going. These psychological factors cannot be underestimated.

> *Use this book as a guide then start experimenting with different foods and fluids throughout training sessions. Discover for yourself what feels most comfortable and works best for you.*

EATING FOR COMPETING: CARBOHYDRATE LOADING – WHAT A LOAD OF GLYCOGEN!

Carbohydrate (or glycogen) loading increases the body's store of glycogen in the liver and muscles. The extra glycogen provides additional fuel for endurance exercise where a normal glycogen store will not be sufficient to maintain stamina.

Early loading methods included a glycogen depletion phase which was employed to make the muscles 'hungry' for glycogen. These early regimens were like torture, as athletes felt tired, irritable and had difficulty maintaining motivation and concentration. After 2–3 days of the depletion phase, a high carbohydrate diet providing 9–10 g of carbohydrate for every kilogram of body weight was consumed for a further 3 days. During this time glycogen stores increased by 200–300 per cent.

In recent times, a modified carbohydrate loading regimen has been developed that results in a similar glycogen store without the unpleasant 'depletion' phase. Athletes simply taper training in the week prior to competition and consume a high carbohydrate diet as described above for 2–3 days prior to competition.

DO YOU NEED TO CARBOHYDRATE LOAD?

All athletes need an adequate normal store of carbohydrate to maximise performance. Carbohydrate loading, in its true sense, is only needed for endurance athletes exercising for greater than 120 minutes in duration e.g. those competing in sports like triathlon, marathon running or ironman events.

WHAT ABOUT THE G.I. AND CARBOHYDRATE LOADING?

At present there is insufficient scientific evidence to recommend a particular G.I. for carbohydrate loading. It appears that high G.I. diets may result in higher muscle glycogen levels in non athletes. It would seem reasonable to propose that a higher G.I. diet may facilitate more effective glycogen loading, but further research is needed.

Carbohydrate loading increases
the body's store of glycogen.
This helps prevent fatigue
in endurance events.

THE PRE-COMPETITION MEAL

The pre-competition meal has the potential to either make or break your performance on the day. What you eat should not be left to chance. Work on a dietary strategy using the following guidelines, then practise this strategy before a training session so you can fine tune your pre-competition meal.

Guidelines

- Eat 2–4 hours before the event. This allows time for your pre-competition meal to be emptied from the stomach. Allow 4 hours for a larger meal.
- Make the meal high in carbohydrate for maximum energy.
- Top up, do not over eat. Eat a comfortable amount of food.
- Keep the fat down in this meal. Fat slows digestion.
- Moderate protein. Fill up on carbohydrates instead.
- Moderate fibre. Too much high fibre food could cause bloating, diarrhoea and be uncomfortable during the competition. Leave your high-fibre eating for non-competition days

- Drink your meal. If you're too nervous, or you feel it's too early in the morning to eat, try a sports drink or liquid meal type drink so that you can maintain your energy with liquid food.
- Practise. Experiment with different meals to find out what works best for you.

ON YOUR MARK
Remember, the pre-event meal won't work miracles if your training diet is inadequate. Make sure you are eating well generally, especially for the week leading up to competition.

GET SET
Use these pre-competition guidelines to help you plan your pre-event meal.

GO
During exercise, replace fluids and carbohydrates regularly as you go.

THE CASE FOR LOW G.I. FOODS

THE PRE-EVENT MEAL

Researchers at the University of Sydney have found that a low G.I. pre-event meal, at least 1 hour prior to endurance exercise, can delay fatigue by delivering greater amounts of carbohydrate to the muscle late in exercise. If you think about it, the low G.I. meal will still be digesting during the exercise session and providing an additional source of carbohydrate that you had long forgotten about. Slow-release (low G.I.) carbohydrate is thought to be particularly useful for exercise of long duration where glycogen stores become limiting.

Athletes like to eat foods that won't be too heavy or fibrous. Before the event, choose low G.I. foods that are not too fibrous or 'gas producing' – taking a 'pit stop' at the loo during exercise can be very inconvenient! Suitable light and low G.I. foods include pasta, some varieties of rice (Basmati), low G.I. breads (those with barley or wholegrains) and some breakfast cereals (e.g. porridge).

If you participate in prolonged (>2 hours) exercise, try a low G.I. pre-event meal to see if this works for you.

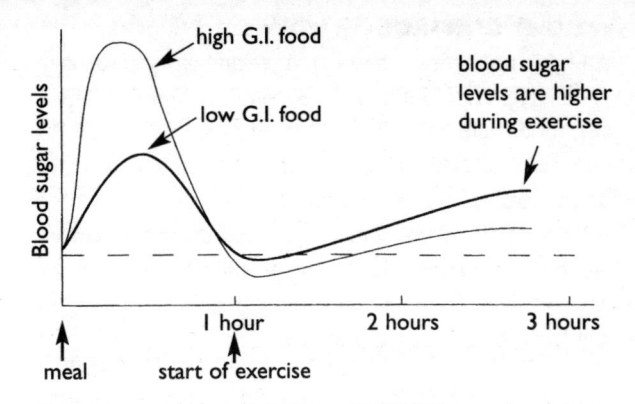

Figure 2. Comparison of the effect of low and high G.I. foods on blood sugar levels during prolonged strenuous exercise. When a pre-event meal of lentils (low G.I. factor) was compared with potatoes (high G.I. factor), cyclists were able to continue cycling at a high intensity (65 per cent of their peak aerobic capacity) for 20 minutes longer after eating the lentil meal. Their blood sugar and insulin levels were significantly higher at the end of exercise, indicating that carbohydrate was still being absorbed from the small intestine even after 90 minutes of strenuous exercise.

WEIGHT CONTROL

A high carbohydrate, low G.I. diet can help you manage your weight and body fat levels with greater ease. Low G.I. foods help you fill up more easily which is useful if you need to control your food intake to stay lean or make a weight for competition.

Fatty foods, in particular have only a weak effect on satisfying appetite relative to the number of Calories they provide. Carbohydrate foods generally make you feel fuller than fats and are far less fattening!

In studies at the University of Sydney, people were given a range of foods that contained an equal number of Calories, then their satiety (feeling of fullness and satisfaction after eating) responses were compared. High carbohydrate, low G.I. foods were more filling and satisfying.

If you need to increase your food intake to gain lean body mass (muscle), excessive amounts of low G.I. food may be just too filling. In this case, you need to balance the G.I. in your meals so you can consume enough food (see Nathan's case history pages 51–53).

COUNTING THE CALORIES IN OUR NUTRIENTS

All foods contain Calories. Of all the nutrients in food that we consume, fat yields the most Calories per gram.

carbohydrate	4 Calories per gram
protein	4 Calories per gram
alcohol	7 Calories per gram
fat	9 Calories per gram

Low fat, low G.I. carbohydrate foods help you to feel full and more satisfied after eating.

THE CASE STUDIES

The following case studies will help you understand the principles of sports nutrition in action. Each case presents common problems or questions and provides simple, practical solutions.

Use this book and others recommended on page 95 to help you plan a better diet to boost your own sports performance. If you get stuck, don't be afraid to seek professional help from a dietitian who is trained to plan out a diet for your specific needs.

Remember, these cases are to be used as a guide only. It is best if you can use the general principles to discover what works best for you.

GO FOR IT!

NATHAN – AUSTRALIAN RULES FOOTBALL

Nathan is an 18-year-old Australian Rules football player. He recently moved from a small country town to take up a position in one of the best sides in the league. Playing professional footy was Nathan's dream. Wanting to make a big impression during his first few weeks at training, Nathan gave his all. At first he felt fine, but after one week of training twice almost every day he felt exhausted, and was frankly 'off the pace'. Sensing that Nathan was struggling, the coach took him aside and recommended he speak to the club's sports dietitian about his diet and recovery strategies.

Nathan's Weekly Training Program
Morning weight/circuit training:
2–3 sessions per week of 1–1.5 hours
Afternoon football/fitness sessions:
4 sessions of 2–2.5 hours per week

Consultation with the sports dietitian

Nathan was a bit wary, he wondered what diet could really do for him. The dietitian explained that carbohydrates were the key to energy and recovery. His diet at the moment was far too low in carbohydrate to get him through the tough pre-season training. The dietitian also explained that eating carbohydrate regularly was important, and fuelling up immediately (within 30 minutes) after training sessions helped to replace the body's carbohydrate stores more quickly. Timing was important because between morning and afternoon training his body had less than 6 hours to refuel. More rapidly absorbing carbs or those with an intermediate to high G.I. were also better for refuelling as they replenished the body's carbohydrate or glycogen levels faster.

The dietitan also explained that to help Nathan maintain his body weight and stay lean he should:

- use lean meats or cut off the fat
- remove chicken skin from chicken
- use reduced fat dairy products
- minimise use of oils, butter or margarine

High G.I. fuel to the rescue
Nathan noticed the other players in his team were already consuming sports drinks with glucose (high G.I.) to begin the refuelling and rehydration process straight after training and chose intermediate to high G.I. breads, cereals or fruit to boost their recovery (French bread, Weetabix, pineapple, watermelon). These foods were available at training so he could

start the refuelling process before travelling home.

The dietitian also organised cooking classes to give him confidence preparing different carbohydrate-based meals for himself. But Nathan now knew that when recovery time was short, higher G.I. carbohydrate meals were best.

Results

Nathan noticed the difference in his performance after being on the high carbohydrate diet for only a few days. He felt fresher at afternoon training and could really power through the sprint sessions which had been like torture before. Including more carbohydrate in his diet and refuelling with higher G.I. carbohydrates really helped him. He knew he still had a lot of work to do before the competition season kicked off but with the right fuel, a great attitude and some raw talent he reckoned he was ready for some of his best ever performances.

MEAL PLAN FOR NATHAN

Aim: To provide sufficient carbohydrate and energy and to assist recovery rate by incorporating high G.I. liquids and intermediate-to-high G.I. meals after training.

8.30 am Immediately post training
1 litre sports/electrolyte drink

9.00 am Breakfast:

1 piece of fruit
2 cups of cereal
2 cups of reduced fat milk
2 slices white or wholemeal
toast (no butter)
with honey
1 glass of fruit juice

Post training
Intermediate to high G.I. choices

Pineapple, Watermelon
Puffed wheat, Weetabix,

White or wholemeal with a
high G.I. (see tables)
French bread has a high G.I.
Pineapple is his favourite juice

11.30 am Snack
1 sandwich (no butter) lean meat filling
1 piece of fruit (any type)
1 low fat yoghurt

1.00 pm Lunch
3 salad sandwiches or rolls filled with
any of the following: lean meat, chicken
reduced fat cheese, egg, canned tuna
in spring water or canned salmon
2 pieces of fresh fruit (any type)
600 ml of reduced fat, flavoured milk

2.30 pm Snack	**Intermediate to high G.I. choices**
Fruit smoothie or a liquid meal	

3.30-5.30 pm Pre- and during training
2–3 litres of sports/electrolyte drink — High G.I. (73–78)

5.30 pm After training:
1 litre sports/electrolyte drink or carb loader — High G.I. for recovery

7 pm Dinner
Large serving lean meat (155 g), or skinless chicken (185 g), or fish (250 g) – grilled or cooked with minimum oil
Large serving of rice, or pasta or potato — High G.I. rice on training nights, pasta most others
Medium serving of vegetables or tossed green salad (no-oil dressing)
4 slices of white bread or 2 rolls (no butter) — High G.I. French bread on training nights

9.00 pm Snack
2 pieces of fresh fruit in a smoothie or fruit and yoghurt

Dietary analysis

Energy:	4480 Calories
Protein:	194 g (17 per cent)
Fat:	67 g (14 per cent)
Carbohydrate:	775 g (69 per cent)

ANALISE – BALLET DANCER

Analise, a 16-year-old full-time ballet student, had a dream: to be a dancer with the Australian Ballet Company. When she started to mature at 13, she found she could no longer 'eat anything' as she used to. Extra weight started to pile on. First she tried all the diets given to her by the other ballet students, but she always felt hungry and craved chocolate. Getting nowhere fast by herself, her mother took her to see a sports dietitian.

Consultation with the sports dietitian

At their first meeting the dietitian took a history of Analise's weight and eating patterns and found that a typical day's meals for Analise included:

A slice of white toast with butter and a cup of strong black tea for breakfast

2 crispbreads with butter and a cup of black tea for a morning snack

A green salad, an apple and a cup of black tea for lunch

A chocolate bar and a can of diet cola during the afternoon (waiting at the train station)

Steamed vegetables, sometimes steamed chicken and a cup of black tea for dinner

A chocolate bar or chocolate biscuits and tea for supper.

The dietitian explained that this diet was high in fat and too low in protein, carbohydrate, calcium and iron. She explained that:

- Gaining a little body weight and fat is part of the maturation process and that the best way to control body fat was with a sensible diet, not starving.
- Cravings are to be expected when you are hungry. After working hard in class all day with virtually no food, chocolate is just too tempting. Eating more carbohydrate on a regular basis would help Analise control her chocolate cravings.
- Analise needed a dietary strategy to give her sufficient fuel to get through the day without feeling hungry. Carbohydrates (especially chrunchy and chewy carbs with a low G.I.) would help her to feel fuller (satiety), give her more energy and are much less fattening than fats. Analise's meal plan, based on reducing fat intake and boosting carbohydrate, meant eating more pasta, rice, bread, fruit and vegetables and less high fat food like butter and chocolate. Chocolate was not totally out but she had to cut back to get her body fat levels going in the right direction. The dietitian also explained that drinking less tea would help Analise maintain adequate iron levels. The tannin in tea reduces iron absorption.

Analise had some questions about the meal plan.

Could she really lose weight eating this much?
The dietitian explained that the size or appearance of foods is often deceiving. Although some high fat foods like chocolate look compact, and foods like bread and vegetables may take up more space on the plate, the fat and Calorie value of high fat foods is much more than bread and vegetables. The fat figures in the back of this book were a real surprise to Analise as was the fact that the fat we eat is converted into body fat, faster and easier than anything else we eat.

Should she cut out chocolate all together?
The dietitian explained that giving up chocolate is really not necessary and is almost impossible unless you live somewhere where there's no chocolate at all. Eating chocolate as a treat rather than a substitute meal is the key.

How could she avoid feeling too full and having a bloated stomach during class?

Foods with a high fibre content (including many salad vegetables) may produce more gas in the intestine and this can cause bloating. The dietitian showed how Analise could increase the intake of low G.I. carbohydrate foods through the day without bloating.

Results

At first Analise kept thinking that she was eating too much. But she found avoiding the chocolate vending machine on the station platform on the way home easier when she felt fuller through the day, the high carbohydrate, low G.I. foods really reduced her hunger. Her body fat level (measured with skinfold callipers) dropped steadily each week. It was almost unbelievable to be able to drop fat without starving. An added bonus was her improved energy levels and concentration in class, not to mention her mood which was more relaxed and cheerful.

ANALISE'S MEAL PLAN

Aim: To provide a regular supply of carbohydrate, with less fat. The G.I. to be intermediate to low to assist with satiety.

8.00 am Breakfast	**Intermediate to low G.I.**
1 piece of fruit	Fresh apple, grapefruit, kiwi fruit
1 cup bran type cereal	All-Bran, oats
1 slice wholegrain toast (no butter) and jam	Oat, barley, mixed grain or fruit breads
1 cup decaffeinated coffee	

10.30 am Snack

1 piece of fruit or a low fat fruit yoghurt

Fruit like, apricot, cherries, orange

1.00 pm Lunch

1 sandwich (no butter). Protein options include: chicken, turkey, canned tuna in brine or water, salmon, reduced fat cheese, lean ham, corn beef or roast meat. Small amount of salad

Oat, barley or heavy grain bread

1 piece of fruit

Peach, pear or plum

Water or a low Calorie drink (not containing caffeine)

3.30 pm Snack

1 raisin toast with jam or ½ muffin with jam.
Or fruit or low fat yoghurt as in morning snack

Raisin bread or grain muffin

7.00 pm Dinner   **Intermediate to low G.I.**

Small serving of lean meat (90 g),
or skinless chicken (125 g) or
grilled fish (155 g).
All cooked in minimum to no oil.

2 potatoes or pasta   New boiled potatoes, pasta
or Basmati rice   Basmati rice

Large serving of vegetables
or salad with low oil dressing
Water or low Calorie cordial

9.30 pm Supper
1 glass of reduced fat milk
1 slice raisin toast with jam

Dietary analysis

Energy:	1300 Calories
Protein:	80 g (24 per cent)
Fat:	20 g (14 per cent)
Carbohydrate:	208 g (62 per cent)
Calcium	800 mg (equal to the recommended daily intake)
Iron	14–18 mg (above the recommended daily intake)

IAN – IRONMAN TRIATHLETE

Ian is a 26-year-old physical education teacher and keen triathlete. He has competed in the Olympic distance for the past 5 years but is now keen to qualify for the ironman triathlon in Hawaii. Ian wanted everything to be spot on for his first ironman race so he could qualify for Hawaii. He approached a sports dietitian to help him plan his dietary strategy and brought a list of questions to ask.

How much carbohydrate does he need in his training diet?

The approximate amount of carbohydrate Ian needs is calculated by multiplying his weight by the carbohydrate requirement appropriate for his activity level.

Ian's weight	75 kg
Approximate carbohydrate requirement for his activity level (see page 21)	8 g/kg
Daily carbohydrate needs for training	75 x 8 = 600 g

This amount of carbohydrate may be too difficult to achieve with food. Liquid carbohydrate supplements like sports drinks can help boost carbohydrate intake.

Ian's Training Program

	AM Training	PM Training
Monday	3 km swim	Track session + 15 km run
Tuesday	3 km swim	100 km cycle
Wednesday	Rest	15 km run
Thursday	3 km swim	100 km cycle
Friday	3 km swim	50 km easy cycle
Saturday	150 km cycle	3 km swim
Sunday	Rest	30 km run

Ian's Vital Statistics
Height 178 cm
Weight 75 kg (has lost 4 kg over the past 3 months)
Sum of 8 skinfolds 50 mm (indicates that Ian is very lean)

How can he incorporate the G.I. into his training diet?

Ian can incorporate the G.I. in his diet mainly by including high G.I. drinks (e.g. sports drinks) during and after training. Intermediate to high G.I. foods after training also help to speed up recovery. At other times, the most important thing is to eat sufficient carbohydrate, whatever the G.I. (Most athletes requiring the amount of carbohydrate that Ian does will feel more comfortable with moderate to lower fibre carbohydrate choices (e.g. white bread, white rice and pasta instead of the wholegrain varieties). Otherwise the sheer volume of the carbohydrate and fibre becomes too bulky and bloating.

Why was he so fatigued lately?
Fatigue is a generalised symptom that has numerous causes. Dietary factors that should be considered include:

- Low iron intake. If this is low, then increased amounts of high iron foods need to be included in the diet. Iron deficiency even in athletes with adequate iron intake does occur, and is more common in endurance athletes.
- Inadequate carbohydrate intake. Fatigue can be experienced if muscle glycogen stores are low indicating inadequate intake of carbohydrate over the day. Tiredness can also be due to low blood sugar. This may occur if there is a long period between meals. Low blood sugar (hypoglycaemia) commonly occurs in early morning or afternoon training sessions where insufficient carbohydrate is consumed before the session.

■ Overtraining is a common problem with endurance athletes. Training programs need to be tailored to the individual, incorporating their personal needs for sleep and taking into account their occupational demands.

Viral illness and a number of other medical conditions are also potential causes of fatigue. Ian would benefit from a referral to a sports physician and an exercise scientist to investigate which factors in particular are causing his fatigue.

Does he need to glycogen load prior to the event?
Since the event will be longer than 2 hours (about 11 hours actually), yes! The meal plan outlines how he can glycogen load using the modified regimen. This regimen involves tapered training and a high carbohydrate diet 3–4 days prior to the race. The diet should provide about 9–10 g of carbohydrate per kg of body weight. Check the meal plan for guidance.

What would be the best pre-event meal?
Ian would benefit from trying a low G.I. meal in practice to see how this worked for him. To maintain gastric comfort, the best low G.I. options would include lower fibre choices such as, white pasta, rolled oats, or a liquid low fat milk based meal.

How could he maintain energy throughout the event?
During the event, maintaining energy and hydration will be a major factor influencing his performance. Sports drinks would be the best option to replace energy and fluids during the race. As sports drinks have a high G.I, they will be a rapidly absorbed and easily available source of carbohydrate. Other high G.I. options include jelly beans, honey sandwiches on high G.I. white bread. As Ian will only be able to carry a small amount of the high G.I. food options, the sports drink will probably provide the basis of his refuelling strategy with foods offering minor support.

To prevent boredom and as a morale booster some of the other offerings at the aid stations (choc chip cookie, jam sandwich, cola drink) could be included in smaller quantities as treats. These provide more of a psychological incentive than physiological boost. Although a little caffeine in the cola drink may help with fatigue later in the race due to its stimulant properties, Ian needs to limit caffeine ingestion to avoid problems with its dehydrating effect and slower stomach emptying which may compromise hydration. Caffeine is also subject to sports drug testing.

IAN'S MEAL PLAN

Aim: To provide sufficient carbohydrate and nutrition for peak performance. The meal plan should include intermediate to high G.I. meals or snacks after training sessions to help maximise the rate of glycogen replacement.

Regular training	Notes on G.I. Intermediate to high G.I. Post training	Loading phase
Breakfast 1–2 pieces of fresh fruit 2 cups cereal 1 cup reduced fat milk 3 slices of toast with honey (no butter) 500 ml fruit juice	Pineapple, watermelon Weetabix, Puffed Wheat High G.I. bread e.g. regular white bread Pineapple	Same breakfast
Snack 1 banana and honey roll 1 glass (250 ml) juice (any type)		As for training plan but add in an additional banana roll or a healthy fruit muffin
Lunch 3 sandwiches with salad (including cheese, chicken, lean meat, egg, tuna or salmon as fillings) 1 piece fruit 1 glass sports drink		Same lunch but add in a honey or jam sandwich for extra carbohydrate
Snack As for morning tea or a fruit smoothie Before and during training Sports drink (volume dependent on session type and duration)		Use a liquid meal carbohydrate or loader. Ensure adequate fluid replacement

Regular training	Notes on G.I. Intermediate to high G.I. Post training	Loading phase

Dinner

Medium serving of lean meat (125g), skinless chicken (155 g), fish (200 g) or a vegetarian meal		Same dinner
Large serving of potato, rice or pasta	High G.I. rice, great after hard afternoon training sessions	
Medium serving of vegetables or tossed green salad, no-oil dressing.		
4 slices of bread or two rolls	High G.I. bread	
2 pieces of fresh fruit	Pineapple, watermelon	
1 glass (250 ml) juice (any)		

Supper

4 pieces raisin toast with jam or honey		Add in a carb-loader drink or a liquid meal
1 glass fruit juice		

Dietary analysis (training)
Energy: 3977 Calories
Protein: 179 g (18 per cent)
Fat: 85 g (19 per cent)
Carbohydrate: 624 g (63 per cent)

Dietary analysis (loading)
Energy: 4500 Calories
Protein: 195 g (17 per cent)
Fat: 85 g (16 per cent)
Carbohydrate: 745 g (67 per cent)

THE PRE-EVENT MEAL PLAN FOR IAN

This meal should be consumed about 2–3 hours prior to competition. Ian had tried out the low G.I. meal in training and wanted to use it in competition. The meals he found most comfortable included:

- Liquid meal plus a serving of stewed apple G.I. = 39
- Rolled oats with skimmed milk and orange juice G.I. = 44
- Tinned spaghetti on grain bread toast G.I. = 47

Results

Ian went on to qualify for Hawaii. Being prepared for this race was crucial to best performance. The Hawaii Ironman was 'awesome' – one of his best-ever life experiences made more enjoyable by being well prepared and well fuelled.

YOUR G.I. QUESTIONS ANSWERED

What should be the overall G.I. of an athlete's diet?

This is a good question and one the scientists are yet to answer. There is evidence that diets with a higher G.I. increase the glycogen storage in the muscle of sedentary individuals. This may help athletes to store glycogen more effectively on a day to day basis. A high G.I. has been shown to enhance the rate of recovery of muscle glycogen after exercise. During exercise, a high G.I. is required to provide a rapidly available fuel source.

I am a recreational jogger, what should be the G.I. of my overall diet?

If the exercise is undertaken as part of a weight loss program, there may be some benefit in choosing low G.I. carbohydrates at each meal for their high satiety value. In general for recreational joggers, it is important to have sufficient carbohydrate in the diet for good health and energy. Since the time to restore glycogen after a work out is likely to be longer than for elite athletes, there is less need to have high G.I. carbohydrates immediately after exercise.

What about the pre-event meal before high intensity or non-endurance exercise?

As mentioned there is evidence that low G.I.

carbohydrates before endurance exercise may help to enhance performance. Studies on shorter term exercise have not been done so we again need to await further research. At this stage, there are many factors to consider in planning an optimal pre-event meal. The timing, the fibre content so as to prevent bloating, the fat content and of course the G.I. Much of the advice about pre-event eating has come from practical experience, and surprisingly little from scientific research. As so many factors need to be considered, the best advice for shorter term exercise at present is for individuals to consider the list of optimal pre-event eating strategies and experiment with foods or meals to determine what works best for them.

What about eating between heats and trials over the day?

There is insufficient scientific evidence to recommend a particular G.I. between events at present. However, it makes sense to include carbohydrates that are rapidly absorbed (i.e. higher G.I.) on a regular basis over the day. Eat little and often. Maintain fluid intake to optimise hydration. In shorter (<1 hour) breaks, rapidly absorbed liquids are probably best. In longer breaks, small, low fat, high carb snacks (e.g. rice cakes, soft fruits, honey sandwiches, sports bars etc.) are recommended.

HOW TO USE THE G.I. TABLES

These simplified tables are an A to Z listing of the G.I. factor of foods commonly eaten in Britain and the Republic of Ireland. Approximately 300 different foods are listed. They include some new values for foods tested only recently.

The G.I. value shown next to each food is the average for that food using glucose as the standard, i.e., glucose has a G.I. value of 100, with other foods rated accordingly. The average may represent the mean of 10 studies of that food world wide or only 2 to 4 studies. In a few instances, British data are different to the rest of the world and we show our data rather than the average. Rice and porridge fall into this category.

We have included some foods in the list which are not commonly eaten (gram dahl) and other foods which may be encountered on overseas trips (e.g. some processed breakfast cereals).

To check on a food's G.I., simply look for it by name in the alphabetic list. You may also find it under a food type – fruit, biscuits.

Included in the tables is the carbohydrate (CHO) and fat content of a sample serving of the food. This is to help you keep track of the amount of fat and carbohydrate in your diet. Refer to pages 18 and 10 for advice on how much carbohydrate and fat is recommended.

Remember when you are choosing foods, the G.I. factor isn't the only thing to consider. In terms of your blood sugar levels you should also consider the amount of carbohydrate you are eating. For your overall health the fat, fibre and micronutrient content of your diet is also important. A dietitian can guide you further with good food choices.

If you can't find a G.I. value for a food you eat on many occasions please email us and we'll give you an estimated value of the food and endeavour to test its G.I. in the future. Address your message to:

j.brandmiller@biochem.usyd.edu.au

The G.I. values in these tables are correct at the time of publication. However, the formulation of some commercial foods can change and the G.I. may be altered. Check our web page for revised and new data.
www.biochem.usyd.edu.au/~jennie/GI/glycemic_index.html

A-Z OF FOODS WITH G.I. FACTOR, PLUS CARBOHYDRATE & FAT COUNTER

Food	G.I.	Fat	CHO (grams per serving)
All Bran™, 40 g	42	1	22
Angel food cake, 30 g	67	trace	17
Apple, 1 medium, 150 g	38	0	18
Apple juice, unsweetened, 250 ml	40	0	33
Apple muffin, 1, 80 g	44	10	44
Apricots, fresh, 3 medium, 100 g	57	0	7
canned, light syrup, 125 g	64	0	13
dried, 5–6 pieces, 30 g	31	0	13
Bagel, 1 white, 70 g	72	1	35
Baked beans, canned in tomato sauce, 120 g	48	1	13
Banana cake, 1 slice, 80 g	47	7	46
Banana, raw, 1 medium, 150 g	55	0	32
Barley, pearled, boiled, 80 g	25	1	17
Basmati white rice, boiled, 180 g	58	0	50
Beetroot, canned, drained, 2–3 slices, 60 g	64	0	5
Bengal gram dhal, 100 g	54	5	57
Biscuits			
Digestives, plain, 2 biscuits, 30 g	59	6	21

Food	G.I.	Fat	CHO
		(grams per serving)	
Biscuits (*continued*)			
Milk Arrowroot, 2 biscuits, 16 g	63	2	13
Morning Coffee, 3 biscuits, 18 g	79	2	14
Oatmeal, 3 biscuits, 30 g	54	6	19
Rich Tea, 2 biscuits, 20 g	55	3	16
Shortbread, 2 biscuits, 30 g	64	8	19
Vanilla wafers, 6 biscuits, 30 g	77	5	21
Wheatmeal, 2 biscuits, 16 g	62	2	12
see *also* Crackers			
Black bean soup, 220 ml	64	2	82
Black beans, boiled, 120 g	30	1	26
Black gram, soaked and boiled, 120 g	43	1	16
Blackbread, dark rye, 1 slice, 50 g	76	1	21
Blackeyed beans, soaked, boiled, 120 g	42	1	24
Blueberry muffin, 1, 80 g	59	8	41
Bran			
Oat bran, 1 tablespoon, 10 g	55	1	7
Rice bran, extruded, 1 tablespoon, 10 g	19	2	3
Bran Buds™, breakfast cereal, 30 g	58	1	14

Food	G.I.	Fat	CHO
			(grams per serving)
Bran muffin, 1, 80 g	60	8	34
Breads			
Dark rye, Blackbread, 1 slice, 50 g	76	1	21
Dark rye, Schinkenbröt, 1 slice, 50 g	86	1	22
French baguette, 30 g	95	1	15
Fruit loaf, heavy, 1 slice, 35 g	47	1	18
Gluten-free bread, 1 slice, 30 g	90	1	14
Hamburger bun, 1 prepacked bun, 50 g	61	3	24
Light rye, 1 slice, 50 g	68	1	23
Linseed rye, 1 slice, 50 g	55	5	21
Melba toast, 4 squares, 30 g	70	1	19
Pitta bread, 1 piece, 65 g	57	1	38
Pumpernickel, 2 slices	41	2	35
Rye bread, 1 slice, 50 g	65	1	23
Sourdough rye, 1 slice, 50 g	57	2	23
Vogel's™, Honey & Oat loaf, 1 slice, 40 g	55	3	17
White (wheat flour), 1 slice, 30 g	70	1	15
Wholemeal (wheat flour), 1 slice, 35 g	69	1	14

Food	G.I.	Fat	CHO
			(grams per serving)
Bread stuffing, 60 g	74	5	17
Breadfruit, 120 g	68	1	17
Breakfast cereals			
All-Bran™, 40 g	42	1	22
Bran Buds™, 30 g	58	1	14
Cheerios™, 30 g	74	2	20
Coco Pops™, 30 g	77	0	26
Cornflakes, 30 g	84	0	26
Mini Wheats™ (whole wheat), 30 g	58	0	21
Muesli, toasted, 60 g	43	9	33
Muesli, non-toasted, 60 g	56	6	32
Oat bran, raw, 1 tablespoon, 10 g	55	1	7
Porridge (cooked with water), 245 g	42	2	24
Puffed wheat, 30 g	80	1	22
Rice bran, 1 tablespoon, 10 g	19	2	3
Rice Krispies™, 30 g	82	0	27
Shredded wheat, 25 g	67	0	18
Special K™, 30 g	54	0	21
Sultana Bran™, 45 g	52	1	35
Sustain™, 30 g	68	1	25

Food	G.I.	Fat	CHO
			(grams per serving)
Breakfast cereals (*continued*)			
Weetabix™, 2 biscuits, 30 g	69	1	19
Broad beans, frozen, boiled, 80 g	79	1	9
Buckwheat, cooked, 80 g	54	3	57
Bun, hamburger, 1 prepacked bun, 50 g	61	3	24
Burghul, cooked, 120 g	48	0	22
Butter beans, boiled, 70 g	31	0	13
Cakes			
Angel food cake, 1 slice, 30 g	67	trace	17
Banana cake, 1 slice, 80 g	47	7	46
Flan, 1 slice, 80 g	65	5	55
Pound cake, 1 slice, 80 g	54	15	42
Sponge cake, 1 slice, 60 g	46	16	32
Cantaloupe melon, raw, ¼ small, 200 g	65	0	6
Capellini pasta, boiled, 180 g	45	0	53
Carrots, peeled, boiled, 70 g	49	0	3
Cereal grains			
Barley, pearled, boiled, 80 g	25	1	17
Buckwheat, cooked, 80 g	54	3	57
Burghul, cooked, 120 g	48	0	22
Couscous, cooked, 120 g	65	0	28

Food	G.I.	Fat	CHO
			(grams per serving)
Cereal grains (*continued*)			
Maize			
Cornmeal, wholegrain, cooked, 40 g	68	1	30
Sweet corn, canned, drained, 80 g	55	1	16
Taco shells, 2 shells, 26 g	68	6	16
Millet Ragi, cooked, 120 g	71	0	12
Rice			
Basmati, white, boiled, 180 g	58	0	50
Tapioca (boiled with milk), 250 g	81	10.5	51
Cheerios™, breakfast cereal, 30 g	74	2	20
Cherries, 20, 80 g	22	0	10
Chick peas, canned, drained, 95 g	42	2	15
Chick peas, boiled, 120 g	33	3	22
Chocolate, milk, 6 squares, 30 g	49	8	19
Coco Pops™, breakfast cereal, 30 g	77	0	26
Condensed milk, sweetened, ½ cup, 163 g	61	15	90
Corn bran, breakfast cereal, 30 g	75	1	20
Corn chips, Doritos™ original, 50 g	42	11	33
Cornflakes, breakfast cereal, 30 g	84	0	26

Food	G.I.	Fat	CHO
		(grams per serving)	
Cornmeal (maizemeal), cooked, 40 g	68	1	30
Couscous, cooked, 120 g	65	0	28
Crackers			
Premium soda crackers, 3 biscuits, 25 g	74	4	17
Puffed crispbread, 4 biscuits, wholemeal, 20 g	81	1	15
Rice cakes, 2 cakes, 25 g	82	1	21
Ryvita™, 2 slices, 20 g	69	1	16
Stoned wheat thins, 5 biscuits, 25 g	67	2	17
Water biscuits, 5, 25 g	78	2	18
Croissant, 1	67	14	27
Crumpet, 1, toasted, 50 g	69	0	22
Custard, 175 g	43	5	24
Dairy foods			
Ice cream, full fat, 2 scoops, 50 g	61	6	10
Ice cream, low fat, 2 scoops, 50 g	50	2	13
Milk, full fat, 250 ml	27	10	12
Milk, skimmed, 250 ml	32	0	13

Food	G.I.	Fat	CHO
		(grams per serving)	
Dairy foods (*continued*)			
Milk, chocolate flavoured, low-fat, 250 ml	34	3	23
Custard, 175 g	43	5	24
Yoghurt			
low-fat, fruit, 200 g	33	0	26
low-fat, artificial sweetener, 200 g	14	0	12
Dark rye bread, Blackbread, 1 slice, 50 g	76	1	21
Dark rye bread, Schinkenbröt, 1 slice, 50 g	86	1	22
Digestive biscuits, 2 plain, 30 g	59	6	21
Doughnut with cinnamon and sugar, 40 g	76	8	16
Fanta™, soft drink, 1 can, 375 ml	68	0	51
Fettucini, cooked, 180 g	32	1	57
Fish fingers, oven-cooked, 5 × 25 g fingers, 125 g	38	14	24
Flan cake, 1 slice, 80 g	65	5	55
French baguette bread, 30 g	95	1	15
French fries, fine cut, small serving, 120 g	75	26	49

Food	G.I.	Fat	CHO
			(grams per serving)
Fructose, pure, 10 g	23	0	10
Fruit cocktail, canned in natural juice, 125 g	55	0	15
Fruit loaf, heavy, 1 slice, 35 g	47	1	18
Fruits and fruit products			
Apple, 1 medium, 150 g	38	0	18
Apple juice, unsweetened, 250 ml	40	0	33
Apricots, fresh, 3 medium, 100 g	57	0	7
canned, light syrup, 125 g	64	0	13
dried, 5–6 pieces, 30 g	31	0	13
Banana, raw, 1 medium, 150 g	55	0	32
Cantaloupe melon, raw, ¼ small, 200 g	65	0	10
Cherries, 20, 80 g	22	0	10
Fruit cocktail, canned in natural juice, 125 g	55	0	15
Grapefruit juice, unsweetened, 250 ml	48	0	16
Grapefruit, raw, ½ medium, 100 g	25	0	5
Grapes, green, 100 g	46	0	15

Food	G.I.	Fat	CHO
		(grams per serving)	
Fruits and fruit products (*cont.*)			
Kiwifruit, 1 raw, peeled, 80 g	52	0	8
Lychee, canned and drained, 7, 90 g	79	0	16
Mango, 1 small, 150 g	55	0	19
Orange, 1 medium, 130 g	44	0	10
Orange juice, 250 ml	46	0	21
Pawpaw, ½ small, 200 g	58	0	14
Peach, fresh, 1 large, 110 g	42	0	7
canned, natural juice, 125 g	30	0	12
canned, heavy syrup, 125 g	58	0	19
canned, light syrup, 125 g	52	0	18
Pear, fresh, 1 medium, 150 g	38	0	21
canned in pear juice, 125 g	44	0	13
Pineapple, fresh, 2 slices, 125 g	66	0	10
Pineapple juice, unsweetened, canned, 250 ml	46	0	27
Plums, 3–4 small, 100 g	39	0	7
Raisins, 40 g	64	0	28
Sultanas, 40 g	56	0	30
Watermelon, 150 g	72	0	8
Gluten-free bread, 1 slice, 30 g	90	1	14

Food	G.I.	Fat	CHO
			(grams per serving)
Glutinous rice, white, steamed, 1 cup, 174 g	98	0	37
Gnocchi, cooked, 145 g	68	3	71
Grapefruit juice, unsweetened, 250 ml	48	0	16
Grapefruit, raw, ½ medium, 100 g	25	0	5
Grape Nuts™ cereal, ½ cup, 58g	71	1	47
Grapes, green, 100 g	46	0	15
Green gram dhal, 100 g	62	4	10
Green gram, soaked and boiled, 120 g	38	1	18
Green pea soup, canned, ready to serve, 220 ml	66	1	22
Hamburger bun, 1 prepacked, 50 g	61	3	24
Haricot (navy beans), boiled, 90 g	38	0	11
Honey & Oat Bread (Vogel's™), 1 slice, 40 g	55	3	17
Honey, 1 tablespoon, 20 g	58	0	16
Ice cream, full fat, 2 scoops, 50 g	61	6	10
Ice cream, low-fat, 2 scoops, 50 g	50	2	13
Jelly beans, 5, 10 g	80	0	9
Kidney beans, boiled, 90 g	27	0	18

Food	G.I.	Fat	CHO
		(grams per serving)	
Kidney beans, canned and drained, 95 g	52	0	13
Kiwifruit, 1 raw, peeled, 80 g	52	0	8
Lactose, pure, 10 g	46	0	10
Lentil soup, canned, 220 ml	44	0	14
Lentils, green and brown, dried, boiled, 95 g	30	0	16
Lentils, red, boiled, 120 g	26	1	21
Light rye bread, 1 slice, 50 g	68	1	23
Linguine pasta, thick, cooked, 180 g	46	1	56
Linguine pasta, thin, cooked, 180 g	55	1	56
Linseed rye bread, 1 slice, 50 g	55	5	21
Lucozade ™, original, 1 bottle, 300 ml	95	<1	56
Lungkow bean thread, 180 g	26	0	61
Lychee, canned and drained, 7, 90 g	79	0	16
Macaroni cheese, packaged, cooked, 220 g	64	24	30
Macaroni, cooked, 180 g	45	1	56
Maize			
Cornmeal, wholegrain, 40 g	68	1	30

Food	G.I.	Fat	CHO
		(grams per serving)	
Maize (*continued*)			
Sweet corn, canned and drained, 80 g	55	1	16
Maltose (maltodextrins), pure, 10 g	105	0	10
Mango, 1 small, 150 g	55	0	19
Mars Bar™, 60 g	68	11	41
Melba toast, 4 squares, 30 g	70	1	19
Milk, full fat, 250 ml	27	10	12
Milk, skimmed, 250 ml	32	0	13
chocolate flavoured, 250 ml	34	3	23
Milk, sweetened condensed, ½ cup, 160 g	61	15	90
Milk Arrowroot biscuits, 2, 16 g	63	2	13
Millet, cooked, 120 g	71	0	12
Mini Wheats™ (whole wheat) breakfast cereal, 30 g	58	0	21
Morning Coffee biscuits, 3, 18 g	79	2	14
Muesli bars with fruit, 30 g	61	4	17
Muesli, breakfast cereal			
toasted, 60 g	43	9	33
non-toasted, 60 g	56	6	32
Muffins			
Apple, 1 muffin, 80 g	44	10	44

Food	G.I.	Fat	CHO (grams per serving)
Muffins (*continued*)			
Bran, 1 muffin, 80 g	60	8	34
Blueberry, 1 muffin, 80 g	59	8	41
Mung bean noodles, 1 cup, 140 g	39	0	35
Noodles, 2-minute, 85 g packet, cooked	46	16	55
Noodles, rice, fresh, boiled, 1 cup 176 g	40	0	44
Oat bran, raw, 1 tablespoon, 10 g	55	1	7
Oatmeal biscuits, 3 biscuits, 30 g	54	6	19
Orange, 1 medium, 130 g	44	0	10
Orange juice, 250 ml	46	0	21
Orange squash, diluted, 250 ml	66	0	20
Parsnips, boiled, 75 g	97	0	8
Pasta			
Capellini, cooked, 180 g	45	0	53
Fettucini, cooked, 180 g	32	1	57
Gnocchi, cooked, 145 g	68	3	71
Noodles, 2-minute, 85 g packet, cooked	46	16	55
Linguine, thick, cooked, 180 g	46	1	56
Linguine, thin, cooked, 180 g	55	1	56

Food	G.I.	Fat	CHO
		(grams per serving)	
Pasta (*continued*)			
Macaroni cheese, packaged, cooked, 220 g	64	24	30
Macaroni, cooked, 180 g	45	1	56
Noodles, mung bean, 1 cup, 140 g	39	0	35
Noodles, rice, fresh, boiled, 1 cup, 176 g	40	0	44
Ravioli, meat-filled, cooked, 220 g	39	11	30
Rice pasta, brown, cooked, 180 g	92	2	57
Spaghetti, white, cooked, 180 g	41	1	56
Spaghetti, wholemeal, cooked, 180 g	37	1	48
Spirale, durum, cooked, 180 g	43	1	56
Star pastina, cooked, 180 g	38	1	56
Tortellini, cheese, cooked, 180 g	50	8	21
Vermicelli, cooked, 180 g	35	0	45
Pastry, flaky, 65 g	59	26	25
Pawpaw, raw, ½ small, 200 g	58	0	14
Pea and ham soup, canned, 220 ml	66	2	13

Food	G.I.	Fat	CHO
		(grams per serving)	
Peach, fresh, 1 large, 110 g	42	0	7
canned, natural juice, 125 g	30	0	12
canned, heavy syrup, 125 g	58	0	19
canned, light syrup, 125 g	52	0	18
Peanuts, roasted, salted, 75 g	14	40	11
Pear, fresh, 1 medium, 150 g	38	0	21
canned in pear juice, 125 g	44	0	13
Peas, green, fresh, frozen, boiled, 80 g	48	0	5
Peas, dried, boiled, 70 g	22	0	4
Pineapple, fresh, 2 slices, 125 g	66	0	10
Pineapple juice, unsweetened, canned, 250 g	46	0	27
Pinto beans, canned, 95 g	45	0	13
Pinto beans, soaked, boiled, 90 g	39	0	20
Pitta bread, 1 piece, 65 g	57	1	38
Pizza, cheese and tomato, 2 slices, 230 g	60	27	57
Plums, 3–4 small, 100 g	39	0	7
Popcorn, low-fat (popped), 20 g	55	2	10
Porridge (made with water), 245 g	42	2	24
Potatoes			
French Fries, fine cut, small serving, 120 g	75	26	49

Food	G.I.	Fat	CHO (grams per serving)
Potatoes (*continued*)			
instant potato	83	1	18
new, peeled, boiled, 5 small (cocktail), 175 g	62	0	23
new, canned, drained, 5 small, 175 g	61	0	20
pale skin, peeled, boiled, 1 medium, 120 g	56	0	16
pale skin, baked in oven (no fat), 1 medium, 120 g	85	0	14
pale skin, mashed, 120 g	70	0	16
pale skin, steamed, 1 medium, 120 g	65	0	17
pale skin, microwaved, 1 medium, 120 g	82	0	17
potato crisps, plain, 50 g	54	16	24
Potato crisps, plain, 50 g	54	16	24
Pound cake, 1 slice, 80 g	54	15	42
Pretzels, 50 g	83	1	22
Puffed crispbread, 4 wholemeal, 20 g	81	1	15
Puffed wheat breakfast cereal, 30 g	80	1	22
Pumpernickel bread, 2 slices	41	2	35

Food	G.I.	Fat	CHO
		(grams per serving)	
Pumpkin, peeled, boiled, 85 g	75	0	6
Raisins, 40 g	64	0	28
Ravioli, meat-filled, cooked, 220 g	39	11	30
Rice			
Basmati, white, boiled, 180 g	58	0	50
Glutinous, white, steamed, 1 cup, 174 g	98	0	37
Instant, cooked, 180 g	87	0	38
Rice bran, extruded, 1 tablespoon, 10 g	19	2	3
Rice cakes, 2, 25 g	82	1	21
Rice Krispies™, breakfast cereal, 30 g	82	0	27
Rice noodles, fresh, boiled, 1 cup, 176 g	40	0	44
Rice pasta, brown, cooked, 180 g	92	2	57
Rice vermicelli, cooked, 180 g	58	0	58
Rich Tea biscuits, 2, 20	55	3	16
Rye bread, 1 slice, 50 g	65	1	23
Ryvita™ crackers, 2 biscuits, 20 g	69	1	16
Sausages, fried, 2, 120 g	28	21	6
Semolina, cooked, 230 g	55	0	17
Shortbread, 2 biscuits, 30 g	64	8	19

Food	G.I.	Fat	CHO
			(grams per serving)
Shredded wheat breakfast cereal, 25 g	67	0	18
Soda crackers, 3 biscuits, 25 g	74	4	17
Soft drink, Coca Cola™, 1 can, 375 ml	63	0	40
Soft drink, Fanta™, 1 can, 375 ml	68	0	51
Soups			
Black bean soup, 220 ml	64	2	82
Green pea soup, canned, ready to serve, 220 ml	66	1	22
Lentil soup, canned, 220 ml	44	0	14
Pea and ham soup, 220 ml	60	2	13
Tomato soup, canned, 220 ml	38	1	15
Sourdough rye bread, 1 slice, 50 g	57	2	23
Soya beans, canned, 100 g	14	6	12
Soya beans, boiled, 90 g	18	7	10
Spaghetti, white, cooked, 180 g	41	1	56
Spaghetti, wholemeal, cooked, 180 g	37	1	48
Special K™, 30 g	54	0	21
Spirale pasta, durum, cooked, 180 g	43	1	56
Split pea soup, 220 ml	60	0	6
Split peas, yellow, boiled, 90 g	32	0	16

Food	G.I.	Fat	CHO
		(grams per serving)	
Sponge cake plain, 1 slice, 60 g	46	16	32
Sports drinks			
Gatorade, 250 ml	78	0	15
Isostar, 250ml	70	0	18
Stoned wheat thins, crackers, 5 biscuits, 25 g	67	2	17
Sucrose, 1 teaspoon	65	0	5
Sultana Bran™, 45 g	52	1	35
Sultanas, 40 g	56	0	30
Sustain™, 30 g	68	1	25
Swede, peeled, boiled, 60 g	72	0	3
Sweet corn, 85 g	55	1	16
Sweet potato, peeled, boiled, 80 g	54	0	16
Sweetened condensed milk, ½ cup, 160 g	61	15	90
Taco shells, 2, 26 g	68	6	16
Tapioca pudding, boiled with milk, 250 g	81	10.5	51
Tapioca, steamed 1 hour, 100 g	70	6	54
Tofu frozen dessert (non-dairy), 100 g	115	1	13
Tomato soup, canned, 220 ml	38	1	15
Tortellini, cheese, cooked, 180 g	50	8	21

Food	G.I.	Fat	CHO
		(grams per serving)	
Vanilla wafer biscuits, 6, 30 g	77	5	21
Vermicelli, cooked, 180 g	35	0	45
Waffles, 25 g	76	3	9
Water biscuits, 5, 25 g	78	2	18
Watermelon, 150 g	72	0	8
Weetabix™ breakfast cereal, 2 biscuits, 30 g	69	1	19
Wheatmeal biscuits, 2, 16 g	62	2	12
White bread, wheat flour, 1 slice, 30 g	70	1	15
Wholemeal bread, wheat flour, 1 slice, 35 g	69	1	14
Yakult, 65 ml serve	46	0	11
Yam, boiled, 80 g	51	0	26
Yoghurt			
low-fat, fruit, 200 g	33	0	26
low-fat, artificial sweetener, 200 g	14	0	12

HOW TO FIND A SPORTS DIETITIAN

■ The best way to obtain the names of sports dietitians practising in your area is to contact:

British Dietetic Association
5th Floor, Elizabeth House
22 Suffolk Street Queensway
Birmingham B1 1LS
Telephone: 0121 616 4900

Irish Nutrition & Dietetic
 Institute
Dundrum Business Centre
Frankfort Dundrum
Dublin 14
Ireland
Telephone: (1)298 7466

■ It is also worth checking in the *Yellow Pages* for your area.

RECOMMENDED READING ON SPORTS NUTRITION

For an expanded discussion on sports nutrition the following books are highly recommended.

Burke L., *The Complete Guide to Food for Sports Performance*, Allen and Unwin 1995

Cardwell G., *Gold Medal Nutrition.*, Glenn Cardwell 1996 (self published)

Garden L., *Footy Food*, Lorna Garden 1993.

O'Connor H and Hay D., *The Taste of Fitness*, JB Fairfax Press 1993

Roberts C and Inge K., *Food for Sport Cookbook*, Rene Gordon 1993

ABOUT THE AUTHORS

Dr Helen O'Connor is a sports dietitian and lecturer in the Department of Exercise and Sport Science at the University of Sydney. Helen consults at the Sydney Sports Medicine Centre, Olympic Park and at the South Sydney Sports Medicine Centre. Academy of Sport. She is the personal dietitian for the Sydney Swans, Canterbury Rugby League and a number of Australia's elite athletes.

Associate Professor Jennie Brand Miller, a member of the teaching and research staff of the Human Nutrition Unit at the University of Sydney, is a world authority on the glycaemic index of foods. Her most recent book was *The Glucose Revolution* (Hodder & Stoughton).

Associate Professor Stephen Colagiuri, Director of the Diabetes Centre and Head of the Department of Endocrinology, Metabolism and Diabetes at the Prince of Wales Hospital, Sydney, has published extensively on carbohydrate in the diet of people with diabetes. His most recent book was *The Glucose Revolution*.

Kaye Foster-Powell, an accredited practising dietitian-nutritionist, is the senior dietitian at Wentworth Area Diabetes Service and conducts a private practice. Her most recent book was *The Glucose Revolution*.